LOSE WEIGHT AND BE FIT NOW

Say No To Snake Oil Weight Loss

Egberto Willies

Email:
egberto@egbertowillies.com

Web:
http://LoseWeightAndBeFitNow.com

Twitter:
http://twitter.com/egbertowillies

My Books:
https://egbertowillies.com/my-books/

CONTENTS

PREFACE

This is a different kind of book for me. I decided to drop what I was writing to write this instead because during and after Christmas I started seeing all those yearly barrages of diet commercials that were taking advantage of both women and men at their most vulnerable time, right after that weight gain from the great holiday feast.

I felt that all the diet commercials were knowingly misleading to do what they do, make a buck on the vulnerable. When will we create laws that prevent these companies from misleading people? We are generally a trusting people and tend to believe that all that we see on infomercials are for the most part truthful. After-all would anyone get on TV, get on the radio, print in newspapers and magazines things that are patently false? The answer is yes. After-all it sure seems that as we get more no-pain weight-loss programs, we are in an ever-expanding weight gain modal.

I have been battling the battle of the bulge for all my life. Inasmuch as many believe that this weight consciousness thing is a woman thing, many of these weight loss companies that market their weight loss snake oil impossibilities strategically cater to both men and women.

I want men and women to see someone, an average person, me, admit to a struggle with weight, admit to the use of many of the snake oils inasmuch as I should have known better, deny the simple arithmetic of weight gain and weight loss, and repeat these shenanigans over and over for decades with no consistent results.

I want those reading this book to see a vulnerable person who finally found a way to succeed in weight loss and fitness. I did not have to buy any pills I did not already buy. I did not have to buy special foods I did not already buy. I did not have to get any special trainers. I just had to do one thing, be honest and be consistent.

It is funny that the most effective way to lose weight and keep it off is to be honest with self. It is not easy, but it is the only thing that can work.

No more going to the restaurant and eating a small meal and finishing my wife's and daughter's plate. No more coming downstairs from my home office and eating a handful of granolas each time. No more eating the bag of potato chips and lying to me about the jaw dropping number of calories in it.

Honesty and acceptance of vulnerability and fallibility made my weight loss program, this time difficult but very successful. This is how I did it. I am sure you can do it either using some of what I did as some sort of inspiration or as a partial guide.

Here is the reality. Do it your way. It works best because once you know the science of weight loss and your own body, your way is the best way for you.

MEA CULPA

Whenever I see a wrong, I am simply wired to speak out in whatever form I have at my disposal, whether it is my own blog, my blogging ring, editorials, or other venues. My belief is that a lot of the weight loss programs out there are morale breakers for many people and should be called out. I think if we all started to feel a bit more responsible for the well-being of our fellow brothers and sisters in the country, we could stop much of the ill doing by many of these snake oil selling entities.

A year and half ago I wrote my first book that did very well "As I See It: Class Warfare the Only Resort To Right Wing Doom" (ISBN: 1-453-60816-8), I started writing my second book about where we must go now in this new economy. It will now be my third book since I decided to put that on hold until I released this one. I figured that I had something to offer that was better for the average person wanting to lose weight than unsustainable and costly options.

I kind of feel guilty about delaying my book on the new economy but writing this book is for me as well. You see, I am at the stage where every so often I want to re-adopt my old habits. Being honest with me as well as being responsible for my written words is yet another tool used to ensure I stay committed to healthy eating as well as weight control and weight maintenance.

I do not write long books. I read a lot of books. Unless the extra fluff is used to add more context and scenery I rather it is left out. It gives me more time to read more books. If I enjoy the book from the author, I would likely purchase another one from him/her as well, especially if it is relatively short.

IN THE BEGINNING

My parents told me that from conception I had a huge appetite. They told me that I would cry until I got that second and third bottle. I was told I was a big baby and the pictures corroborate this. I was big but not obese.

Did I really want a bottle or something else? Was that extra milk just comfort, for some underlying something else? One never knows. After all, toddlers usually can't speak that well to articulate any need particularly. I would wager that that habit of just screaming for the comfort of that bottle and getting it from parents who only wanted me to be calm and happy was the beginning of the weight problem I had.

In my house food was never a problem. There was a lot of it. My mother is the best cook on the planet. Well my wife does an excellent emulation with her own personal twists. And I am not saying this to get in my wife's good graces, but my mom can burn.

To this day every time I spend Christmas with her in California, salivation begins weeks before the trip. I am salivating now thinking about her cooking.

My mother would tell my sisters to eat all the food off their plates. She never had to tell me that (unless it was spaghetti). The staple in my house was rice & beans, chicken, fresh pork, and steak. And I mean daily. A stay home mother can be a clear and present danger to maintaining a healthy weight unless you are predisposed to eating healthy.

In our household unlike most we had the big meal at noon. We went to school from 8 AM to 12 Noon. We came home to eat (this is possible in little towns since it took five to ten minutes or so to get home). She had a full meal sitting at the table by the time we got home. After that complete meal we went back to school till around 5 PM or so.

Then there was the snacking. Any of you remember Big60? It was those cream filled vanilla and chocolate cookies. They imported them from the United States, and it was the snack staple in my house. Every two weeks my parents would go to the grocery store to replenish the supply. And with ample supplies of milk, I had dessert throughout the day.

What am I trying to say? In the beginning there has always been food. Some of us simply eat it incessantly if it is there. Others are simply not interested.

My two sisters were never big eaters like I was and our weight differential was always evident. I was not obese, but I was overweight like most Americans are today.

I had been obese, and I had been extremely thin over the last 35 years. The fact is that I was wrong in how I handled my weight problem. Most of the books I read were wrong not necessarily because they were disingenuous, but because they used our own psychology against us. If we believe something is going to be hard and take a long time we give up.

I am not going to lie to you. I will tell you the different avenues I've taken and then what worked and is working.

In fact, as I am writing this book, I am on the deck of the Carnival Cruise ship Triumph in the middle of the Gulf of Mexico. I am enjoying eating much more than I do at home, but I am exercising every morning as well as doing a lot of walking (more stairs than elevators). I will make up the difference when I get home and calculate how many calories I need to burn from over eating based on my weight gain which should be rather small.

It is important to note that I know I will be having 5 days of overeating. I will reduce my caloric intake **immediately** after the trip because it will be easier and more manageable if I undo a little than to wait until I accumulate several bouts of overeating then trying to undo it all at once later. It is all about discipline.

THE SCIENCE
OF WEIGHT
MANAGEMENT

This will likely be my shortest chapter. I am an engineer and the only thing I believe in absolutely is numbers.

There are only two numbers you need to be sure about. One is a known and the other you must figure out.

The first number you need is the caloric content of fat. There are 3,500 calories in every pound of fat you want to get rid of from your body.

The other number you need to know is how many calories your body expends on an average day. This number is hard to figure out and, in my case, took months to figure out.

What I did is weighed myself every day for a month and counted every calorie I ate for that month. Subtract 3500 for every pound you gained and divide that number by 30. For your lifestyle that is the number of calories needed to maintain your weight.

In my case I can eat 2510 calories with my lifestyle and maintain my weight. Here is how I came up with it. I ate 85,800 calories in 30 days. I gained three pounds in those 30 days.

85,000 minus 10,500 calories (3 pounds of weight gain in calories) divided by 30. That meant I can keep my lifestyle which was moderate exercising and eating my peanut butter every day. I simply love peanut butter.

If you want to take some of that fat off of your body, there are only four ways to do it. Everyone rich or poor can choose three of them.

You can go to a doctor and have them suck the fat out. Without a lifestyle change, that is a temporary fix and can go wrong. It could even be life threatening if done incorrectly.

The other options are eating less, exercising more, or a combination of both. I chose the latter.

Remember the numbers. For every pound you want to lose you must eat 3500 less calories or increase your exercise to burn that much more calories or some combination of the two.

If you have 10 pounds to lose then you must take in 35,000 less calories than your body needs. It sounds insurmountable but it is doable in small steps. I had 35 pounds to lose and I did it in about 4 months. It was not easy. But I followed a path and stuck with it most of the times.

Note that I said I stuck with it most of the times in those four months. I fell off the wagon five or six times in that period, but the thing is if your trend line is toward a change, you will ultimately lose weight.

Remember, it is a lifestyle change that has no end. So, when you screw up you must just call it a day, or a week, or whatever and move on. Do not beat up on yourself as there is no real change in outcome whether you beat up yourself or just get back into forward moving compliance.

MY ART OF WEIGHT OSCILLATION

While I hated my ever-increasing waist-line while in high school, I did nothing about it. I was just a big guy. I was not fat. Really? Yes, I was fat; not obese; but fat.

The reality is when I think back at the volume of food I ate back in Panamá, I fail to see why I was not obese. Then again in those days we did not have video games. In those days we did not spend all day in front of the television or computer as many of the young folks do today.

HIGH SCHOOL

My high school weight was a prelude to things to come, however. I was not overly conscious of it, but it still bothered me that I was bigger than most.

I had severe scoliosis and though big was never athletic. I had surgery to stabilize my scoliosis where a one-foot steel rod was placed on my spine to jack most of the top curvature out. They chiseled bone from my pelvic to fuse five of the curving vertebras into one solid bone.

I was in a body cast for over a year, a painful experience. In that year my muscles in my upper body atrophied to almost skin and bones. After the cast was removed my eating habits were reflected in the growth of my girth.

COLLEGE

I got a 2-year scholarship to go to Blinn College in Brenham Texas in 1979. When I got to Blinn College, I got a job in the school cafeteria. That was the worst thing that could have happened to my weight.

Think about this. A kitchen filled with older southern women that could cook. A green behind the ear foreign student that each one of them thought they needed to mother. These ladies ensured I was fed not only with cafeteria food, but with their delicious soul food they would bring for me all the times.

As I write I remember a funny story. One of my cafeteria-moms asked; Son, do you eat "poe?" I was lost. I told her that I had never heard of "poe." I asked her what "poe" was. She pointed at a pork chop and said, "I know you must eat poe where you from!" "Poe!" "Poe!" A bit embarrassed I said, "I am sorry mam. In Panamá we call it pork" After that I began learning southern English rather quickly.

That cafeteria had a milk dispenser that I had to keep filled with some very large bladders of milk. We had those big plastic 20-ounce cups for drinks. I would drink the milk like it was water. In the mornings I would eat as much bacon and sausage patties I could hold with those delicious southern made hot biscuits.

I was a 6 feet 2 inches 200-pound muscle-less kid when I started Blinn. After a year I weighed in at 265 pounds. Lucky for me, I went to Austin to visit one of my friends at Houston Tillotson College. I visited the campus of the University of Texas at Austin (UT) and fell in love. I knew that I was going to give up my Blinn scholarship because I was going to UT.

In 1980 foreign tuition was 10 times that of in state tuition. In state students paid $4.00 per semester hour while the foreign rate was $40.00 per hour. What did this mean? It meant I had to work my butt off to raise the money to go to UT.

During that summer I got a job at a cotton mill in Brenham. I worked the graveyard shift which was between 11:00 PM to 7:00 AM. I then went to Blinn College to work between 7:00 AM and 11:00 AM in the cafeteria. I slept till around 2:00 PM. I then got up and sold fireworks for the husband of the woman who managed Blinn's cafeteria until around 10:00 PM or so. I then started the cycle all over again.

I worked that schedule for 3 months. Suffice it to say, by the time I started at the University of Texas, I had lost most of the weight. I was somewhere around 210 pounds.

While at the University of Texas, one of my first jobs was a security guard that worked under the campus police. I worked the graveyard shift for about 20 hours a week. The guys would pick me up for a late dinner around 2:00 AM. We would go to a diner that no longer exist on the main campus drag and ate. I fell in love with those southern biscuits and gravy.

As I recall the meal was simply three hot biscuits doused with cups of meaty sausage white gravy. I always ate it all. My weight ballooned back to 245.

By this time, I became very weight conscious because I simply did not feel good or look good. I started playing tennis in the afternoons, mostly with the wall at the university's tennis complex. I would also play with a roommate every so often. I then created my own diet plan. I had a cup of tasteless yogurt for breakfast. In those days there was no Equal nor Splenda sweeteners. All I remember was saccharin and I hated the bitter aftertaste, so my sweet tooth was left unfulfilled. I would have a half head of iceberg lettuce with a can of tuna with tons of garlic powder and a half cup of cottage cheese for dinner. I had the same exact monotonous menu for my diet for three months. I never faltered once. I could be anal back in those days. My wife and daughter may say I am still anal today but that is beside the point.

Within three months I was down to 185 pounds. I don't think I had seen 185 since junior high school. I was very thin but muscle-less at that weight. I felt great, however. I bought all new clothes (on the free-flowing credit all UT students got then and are still getting now). I was paying for those clothes, way after graduation.

WORKING BACHELOR

I held a good weight till I got my first job. After getting my first job I found Dunkin Doughnuts and developed a love affair with their apple fritters. I remember eating six apple fritters for dinner several times a week with several cold beers. You must forgive me. I was a bachelor.

Now while I gained a lot of the weight, because I developed a love for racquetball, my weight simply increased to around 225.

But you know where I am going. I had to lose that weight. I ended my relationship with the Dunkin Doughnut apple fritter and joined the aerobics class at "President's and First Lady" gyms (now Bally's).

There was a lot of incentive for a bachelor like me to attend those classes consistently and lose weight. The classes were filled with beautiful women, none of them overweight. I was one of few men that attended those classes. I do not think it was very macho to do the aerobics thing in the 80s if you were male. I did not care. I got to hug many women as we did the Texas aerobic kick.

I lost all the weight in no time. This time all I did was aerobics every day with peanut butter and jelly sandwiches for breakfast lunch and dinner of course with any light beer I could find.

I got my weight down to a manageable 205 pounds with a better body tone. I kept the weight off for a long time since I did aerobics and racquetball virtually 7 days a week. My bachelor life consisted of work, racquetball, aerobics, partying and developing software in alternate months, trying new businesses, failing at some, and moving from one company to the next. That regime did not leave much time for weight gain.

MARRIED LIFE

Then marriage came and visited me. To put it bluntly, I let myself go. My wife turned into a great cook and it was visible all over my waistline, my face, and my stamina. I ballooned to 250 pounds and stayed there till I had a little scare.

Every time I came out of the shower, I would look at my wife, who was 115 pounds when I met her and asked her if I looked fat. She would constantly tell me that I wasn't. That was my permission slip to keep eating inasmuch as I had eyes and mirrors all over the place that was telling otherwise.

My wife never told me I was busting out of my clothes. She would just buy me more and say the new ones looked better.

After a couple years of marriage, I started my own company and worked from a home office. Of course, that meant the refrigerator and food cabinet was a short distance away and always stocked with food. I made ample use of my legs to get a stack with every refill of my coffee cup.

In those days I drank three to four pots of coffee. That's a whole lot of trips to the kitchen. My trip back from the kitchen included Snickers, potato chips, pretzels, candy, yogurt. It was just eating because it was there.

After my business took off, we moved into a neighborhood with trails. My daughter started elementary school and she went to school through the trails.

I would walk through the trails to pick up my daughter from school every so often. I always walked at a brisk pace irrespective of weight.

One day on my way to pick her up, my heart started beating erratically. This gave me the scare of my life.

I sat down for a while at her school for 20 minutes, but the erratic heart beat continued. I called my wife who picked me up and took me straight to the emergency room.

By the time we got there the heartbeat was normal again. They gave me a 24-hour monitor and found a few irregular beats they did not seem too concerned about. They then did some sort of radiation test that allowed them to see all the arteries and veins in my heart. Everything checked out. My diagnosis was pretty much, lose some weight.

After checking out that my heart was alright, I started back using my dormant for years Bally's membership to get back in shape. I starved myself and worked out like a mad man till I got down to 225 pounds.

I maintained that weight for a few years. At 225 I was not fat, but I always felt I needed to be at a lower weight mostly because the BMI said so.

THE CYCLIST

One afternoon at a PTA function at my daughter's school, her friend's dad asked me if I was interested in cycling with them. I had never cycled in a group but accepted the invite and joined their group. It was the first time I ever did any kind of organized (and expensive) athletic activity. To this day I remember the first day I went out with my broke down bike. One of the guys was bold enough to tell me if I was going to ride with them I needed a real bike. My real bike then was an inexpensive Trek 2200 ($800.00).

We rode a lot including four MS-150 rides which is a 180-mile ride between Houston and Austin. My only goal was to stay on my bike as we entered the steep hills in the hill country entering Austin. I did it. During this I maintained my weight at around 225. Inasmuch as I was riding 200 miles a week in training, I was eating that right back up.

When this group fizzled, I joined another group that was much faster and much more bike conscious. One of the guys tapped me and said, hey man, you need a bike. He volunteered and took me to get an inexpensive higher end bike ($2,500.00 + much more in biking gear for winter and summer).

I burned a ton more calories with this group. On Saturdays and Sundays, we did 60+ miles each day at 21+ miles per hour (sometime sprints of 26 to 29 miles per hour). I did 6 more of those MS-150 180-mile rides between Houston and Austin. We also did several 60+ mile rides in the Texas Hill Country and Houston area flat lands.

During our very active period I probably got down to 220 pounds or so. The point I am making here is that as I exercised more, I simply gave myself permission to eat more. Sometimes more than I worked out.

After doing this for 10 years or so and watching many of my cycling buddies fall and break arms, get concussions, break clavicles, break thumbs, and get hit by cars, I thought that my 10 year virtually accident free period was statistically at risk, so I stopped cycling cold turkey.

THE GYM DAEMON

After I stopped cycling, I knew I had to find some other means of getting exercise. I joined Family Fitness which was closer to my home than Bally's. I kept the Bally's membership since it was really cheap after having it for over 20 years. It cost me about $60.00 a year and if I am out of town, I have a place to work out since it is national. Remember that before you cancel any old memberships.

I worked out for about an hour a day. But if I want to be honest with myself it would be what I call a sedentary workout. The weight lifting did little to build muscle and the aerobics did little to really work up a sweat. But I could tell everyone that I was working out.

Eventually with the constant weight gain I increased the intensity but because I had no plan and continued with my bad eating habits, it was futile. Think about this; it takes me about an hour to burn 900 calories on an elliptical. A Burger King meal (upsized) wipes all of that out plus more. Losing or maintaining weight by exercising alone is impossible.

THE NEW BEGINNING

Up to about 2 years ago my weight started creeping up again till it reached 235. I was feeling that loss of stamina again inasmuch as I was working out relatively hard.

Jim, a friend of mine at the gym challenged me to a weight loss duel. I think the bet was something like $5.00 and bragging rights.

Every Monday we would weigh in. I dreaded it some Mondays because some weekends I did fall off the wagon. Jim won most of the first weeks of our challenge.

I had to get serious about understanding what I knew and putting it into effect not only to make good of Jim's challenge but to make it a long lasting event even after our challenge was done.

Suffice it to say we both lost a lot of weight. After our challenge was up, I decided to continue. I had gotten down to 212 pounds. I wanted to make it to 195. On my birthday, I made it to 193 pounds. Mission accomplished? Not really. The toughest part is how do you keep it off? I will talk about that later.

HOW I LOST THE WEIGHT

It is funny that when Jim made the weight loss challenge in early December, I had already decided that that would be my New Year's resolution. I was turning fifty. I wanted to begin my sixth decade (did I say that?) at the ideal weight for my body type. Fifty was going to be a milestone for me. No more midlife crisis. Midlife was now firmly engrained in my psyche.

When I got back from California, we met at the gym the first day after the New Year and weighed in. I was 235 pounds. I was wearing a size 36/38 pants. My goal was 195 pounds and a size 32 pants.

My 5 day a week routine always involved one hour on the elliptical and about thirty minutes of moderate weight lifting. Since I did that type of working out of course I thought I could eat and snack at will. The progressive weight increase over the years said otherwise.

In effect I was about 35 to 40 pounds overweight. Remembering what I discussed in the section "The Science of Weight Management" I needed to somehow burn 140,000 calories more than I would take in within 4 months to make it by my birthday. It sounds insurmountable but broken down into manageable pieces it is doable.

All the weight loss commercials will tell you that you won't be hungry losing weight. They will also tell you it will be easy. That is simply not true unless you are using some unhealthy appetite suppressant which is unsustainable in the long run. I will be honest. I was hungry a lot and it was hard to be disciplined.

A few weekends into my program I gave in to bodily temptations and did over eat and ate the wrong things. The most important thing however is as opposed to giving up, I continued.

140,000 CALORIES IN 4 MONTHS

But I digress. 140,000 over 120 days (4 months) requires that I eat 1167 calories less than I normally ate even with the exercising that I had been doing. This is not as bad as it seems. I was eating over 3500 calories a day when I count the constant snacking.

Remembering that with my regular moderate exercise I could eat 2500 calories and maintain my weight, I just needed to increase the strenuousness of my exercise to expend more calories and reduce my eating by about 600 calories.

I increased my work out by an extra half an hour. I will be honest. This was extremely hard at first. It got better after a couple of weeks, but it was always strenuous and at the end I was extremely tired even after the body adjusted.

I would only recommend the increase exercise output for those who are very physically fit and have a much higher than average tolerance for pain. As a cyclist that road several sixty to one hundred mile rides several times a week, I knew my body could handle it.

For those folks who are not as physically fit, losing weight over a longer period is likely more do-able and sustainable.

As I mentioned before, I fell off the wagon several times where I went out with the family and over-ate, went out with friends and overate, or simply just stayed home and overate. The most important thing was that I beat up on myself for a few minutes then I continued with the program.

DOCUMENTING, TWITTER, & FACEBOOK

I have a habit of documenting just about everything. I can generally go back and find information on just about every aspect of my life in some one of my databases.

I found that that habit had a lot of value during and after my weight loss program. Many times, when one is dieting or trying to lose weight, it is easy to justify stagnant weight loss as a plateau. The reality is that it is impossible to plateau for an extended amount of time. As an engineer I know that. After all, if you could keep eating fewer calories and still gain or maintain weight in effect you would be creating weight (well mass) out of thin air and that is impossible. The Conservation of Energy and Mass is still valid physics.

The reality is if you are eating fewer calories than you are burning after water retention is considered, your weight must proceed to fall. There is just so much water you can retain after all.

The problem is when we snack or eat a few bites here and there; it is calories we are taking in. Many times, we refuse to take these into account.

I decided to document absolutely everything that I ate. Doing this allowed me to really see what I was eating. You would be surprised how much snacking can contribute to your daily caloric intake.

I found a site that made it easy to document all the food I ate, the calories I burned from exercising, as well as monitoring my weight loss progress.

The site that I used and continue to use is www.myfitnesspal.com. This site made it extremely easy to document all the food that I ate. It also allowed me to document every exercise routine I was doing. It charted my weight and kept my daily caloric intake in a database that I could always go back to.

The best part of www.myfitnesspal.com is that I could access it from my Droid phone, my Xoom pad, or from my desktop. All the data is synced so you can see it all no matter which device you used to enter it. It also encourages including friends or others who can serve as motivators. You can friend me on www.myfitnesspal.com if you need some motivation.

I walk around with my cell phone so as I snacked,

I simply entered the food I ate immediately. What was great is that the site also has a database of thousands of foods so you may not have to figure out the caloric intake yourself.

Doing this type of monitoring ensures that you don't fool yourself about the quantity of food you are eating. To be sure, BS in is equal to BS out. It is important that you are honest with portion sizes that you are entering the application.

You can link your account with your Facebook account and/or your Twitter account. I linked both. What is neat about it is that you can set it up to auto post and auto tweet whenever you post your exercise weight change or when you post a message. You would be amazed at what some of the positive affirmations you get from some of your Twitter and Facebook friends will do to keep you on track.

I remember one Twitter follower had not seen one of my updates for over a week. They summarily sent me a message asking me what was up. I do not know that person personally nor do they know me except as a Twitter exercise buddy. It turned out I was exercising but not recording it and as such not sending tweets on my progress. I immediately started recording again. That is one of the advantages of adding your plan to your social networks. You have a network watching you and keeping you on track.

There are other tools out there, but both my daughter and I have found this particular tool to be very easy to use and conducive to success.

MY EXERCISE ROUTINE

During the four months or so that it took me to lose the 35 to 40 pounds I followed the same routine five days a week. I knew I had to do both aerobics and muscle building.

I packed my gym bag every night before I went to the gym. I woke up at around 4:10 AM Monday through Friday. I would be at the gym by 4:30 AM.

I started with half hour of weightlifting. Following was my routine.

- 2 Sets of 10 Bench press
- 2 Sets of 10 Pectoral
- 2 Sets of 10 Inclined Pectorals
- 2 Sets of 10 Pulls
- 2 Sets of 10 Triceps
- 2 Sets of 10 Pull downs
- 2 Sets of 10 Bicep Curls

I used the just under the heaviest weight I could

do comfortably. Because I did these every day, I made sure to not to do it to the extent to wear out my muscle.

After the weight training I then did one hour on the elliptical machine. I did this at a rather fast pace. I was generally sweating profusely within 10 minutes. Then again, I sweat a lot.

I followed that with a half hour on the same elliptical or a stair step machine. The intensity level here dropped but it still burned enough calories to keep me on track.

After the aerobic exercise I then worked on my abs.

- 2 Sets of 25 on the incline
- 3 Sets of 100 on the horizontal abs machine.

I did that workout for almost four months. There were a few lapses here and there when I had to travel out of town or when I got the flu. I made sure to simply pick up where I left off.

It is always OK to screw up here and there. It is never OK to not jump back into the plan. I believe that is the biggest problem I have had in the past and likely many. If you fall off the wagon, there is no reason to stay off. Staying off, just makes the problem progressively worse.

Now the exercise routine I used to lose weight was aggressive. The fact is that I wanted fast results and remember it started out as a competition. Competing towards a goal can give that extra bit of will power to keep on.

Now I will be honest. I would not advise everyone to do it the way I did it. It was difficult and to be honest, unnecessary. By extending my goal by two months, I could have made my workout routine substantially easier.

In fact, it is best that one works below peak level to maintain consistency. Very hard workouts for most are unsustainable and many times lead to the abandonment of the whole project.

MY DIET

In the section *The Science of Weight Management* I went over the reality about calories. That chapter is one of the most important chapters in this book.

Humans tend to work on gut feelings. Sadly, relying on the gut is generally wrong when interpreting the reality of what we have eaten compared to what we believe we have eaten.

I have read many diet books that claim counting calories is not necessary. I have seen many videos and plans that even discourage counting calories.

Many diet plans will try to draw distinctions between types of calories – eat less carbohydrates – eat less fat – eat more protein. Here is the reality. Calories are the only sure thing you can monitor. No one knows exactly how efficient or inefficient one's body is to the different food types. As such, one should only worry about caloric intake and adjust accordingly to one's basal metabolic rate we previously discussed.

Keep yourself in a fad free zone. A calorie is a calorie is a calorie. Be anal about it. As I mentioned in the section Documenting, Twitter, & Facebook, every calorie eaten was documented on the corresponding app for the myfitnesspal.com. Even if I went to restaurants, I recorded the foods I ate and the quantity.

I did not eat any "diet" foods. I simply reduced my food intake substantially. Yes, I was hungry a lot. Weighing every day and seeing true weight loss every few days made it bearable.

I also made videos cooking foods we all eat in a manner that made it more filling. I also blogged about what I was doing.

I made a lot of stir-fried vegetables, hearty vegetable soups, and many meatless dishes.

A typical breakfast would be a peanut butter sandwich with black coffee and a banana. For lunch I may have a bowl of tomato soup. For dinner I would have stir fry vegetables (a lot). Stir frying cabbage, onions, carrots, parsley, celery, and garlic along with a lot of black pepper and other seasoning makes a tasty meal. What is great is you only need a little bit of olive oil to stir fry a ton of vegetable and it is very filling.

But don't forget, you have got to count those calories; the oil, the vegetables, everything.

There are videos and recipes at this book's website at http://LoseWeightAndBeFitNow.com. Feel free to send me some pictures of your food and recipes and I will post them in your name.

HOW I AM KEEPING THE WEIGHT OFF

The most difficult part after losing weight is keeping most of it off. You will likely put a few pounds on as your body normalizes to an increase in food and likely decline in strenuous exercising.

I went through this. I panicked when I put on a few pounds until I realized what was going on. I was still counting calories and exercising (a bit less) but based on my calculations my weight should have been steady.

Maintaining one's weight is not an exact science and as such while panicking is unnecessary, monitoring one's weight is essential. You should weigh every day, but at least once a week. This will ensure that you can nip any weight increase trend before it gets out of hand.

Most people that gain back their weight or more suffer from not understanding that while incremental weight gain may be small cumulative weight gain occurs from all those daily or weekly incremental weight gains and can get large very fast.

It is for this reason that it is essential that you weight yourself frequently. It is easy to lose a 2-pound weight gain in a week. It is difficult to lose a 10-pound weight gain after a month.

After I reached my ideal weight, I continued to do a very robust exercise program. It was no longer as strenuous as it was during the weight loss stage.

I went from one and a half hours 5 days a week of aerobics to just about one hour 5 days a week. My weight lifting went to around 20 minutes. I still do a lot of abdomen work, but that is not very strenuous.

I watch what I eat. Most importantly I count calories. Yes, I still count calories to ensure I am not eating more than I am burning. Note however that every so often I still over eat. I would go to a restaurant and pig out. That is the reality of life.

When I overeat however, I make sure that I adjust either my future eating or workout regimen to minimize the damage. Once I get back into my weight range, all is normal again.

CONCLUSION

Losing weight is not easy but neither is it diffi-cult. It simply requires that you tell yourself you want to make a change. Assuming you are healthy, do not do it until you are ready. If for medical reasons you must lose the weight now, I am confident using some of my techniques will be useful.

ADDENDUM 2019

I wrote this book in 2013. As I recall, there was much happening with both my software company as well as my ever-increasing political activities. I decided to transition most of my software to a friend's company in New York. He handles all the support and licensing. I could not leave my customers hanging because I wanted to be a small part of making a better country for us all.

I did not publish the book even though it was complete mostly because I was busy doing so many other things. During that time, I've started two other books that I intend to publish this year.

This addendum is necessary. It teaches that humility and fallibility is something we must have when dealing with weight control and many other aspects of our lives.

BACKSLIDING
ONE MORE TIME

I kept the weight off for some time after writing the book. But I lost my way a few years after that. I got back up to 235 ponds.

Lucky for me I did not throw away all my 36 pants, so I did not have to purchase new close for the weight gain. I just quietly slipped into my more comfortable clothes.

It turned out I did not follow one of the important rules I laid out. Weigh consistently and nip any small weight gain immediately.

The truth is, rarely does one need a scale to know when one gains a few pounds. I had to go through the routine I described in this book all over again. But in doing so, I proved that the calculations and techniques were sound.

I lost all the weight again and there are two incentives to keep it off.

MY MOST RECENT MEDICAL SCARE

Please indulge the way I am describing the latest medical scare that made me do the right thing and lose the weight once and for all. I must use it as not only as a reason to lose weight but as an admonition to the sorry state of our healthcare system.

While running the board for the ThinkWing Radio w/Mike Honig Show at KPFT 90.1 FM, a Pacifica radio station in Houston, Texas, I had a potentially fatal blood pressure rise. 244+ over 144+. Yes, those were the actual numbers measured both by the equipment at the station and by the paramedics.

The staff called 911. Some great paramedics came, gave me oxygen, took me into the ambulance, gave me an EKG, and continued to monitor my pressure. It went down some, though still at a dangerous level. When it was time to leave the paramedics asked if I wanted to go to the hospital in the ambulance, which one, or if I wanted to go in my own vehicle. I immediately inferred that they were cognizant that many folks are justifiably concerned about cost.

Since my EKG was perfect and the blood pressure had dropped some, I told them I would drive to an emergency room. My insurance encourages urgent care centers. I drove to a private emergency center not knowing that it wasn't an urgent care center for my medical issue.

The doctor at the ER told me I could have stroked out. He gave me two little pills that dropped the pressure. The doctor asked if I had a headache. I told him I had a slight one. He told me I needed to have a CT Scan. The CT Scan was a newer smaller machine that did the job in less than 5 minutes. I spent less than two hours in an ER mostly waiting for the pressure to fall. I was the only patient in that ER.

After stabilizing my pressure, they told me to see my primary care physician.

The next day my primary care physician was completely booked. Another doctor in the office had an opening but since she was not my primary care physician, I would have needed a referral. After going back and forth with the insurance company and the doctor's office, I got an appointment that would be two days later. They told me if there was an emergency, I should go to the emergency room.

I relayed to the office of my primary care physician with the insurance company on three-way that a system that requires one to go the emergency room not because of lack of capacity or doctors but because of an ill-conceived structure is the problem with our healthcare. An hour later I got a call from the office of my primary care physician to come in.

Since I do not get a subsidy for insurance, I purchased my insurance from a broker. All insurance whether on the Obamacare exchange or elsewhere must have the protections defined in the Affordable Care Act before the Trump administration allowed these companies to start writing inexpensive junk policies again. Sadly, while the safeguards were there, they are useless if you are unable to use the system because of the controls that are clearly designed for profit maximization.

The bill for the CT Scan and the two little pills was $5,000 that I must pay out of pocket. That meant I was out about $10,000 so far that year in health care cost (including insurance premiums). It was a direct transfer of wealth from the middle-class, me, to the stockholders of the private emergency room that took care of me. In health care, there is little ability to shop around during an emergency. Even in non-emergency situations, recent studies suggest consumer shopping around does little to control cost.

I now have two incentives to keep the weight off. The first is that I got rid of all my 34, 36, and 38 clothes. I am stuck with size 32s. The second is encounters with the healthcare system is detrimental to my personal economy.

I am sure we all have incentives to lose weight. Just know we can all make the commitment to do so. There are times we will backslide. But as long as we have more good days than bad ones, we can do just fine.

Positive affirmations.